Delicious Vegetarian Diabetic Meals For One

Polly Fielding

ISBN: 1548789917
ISBN-13: 978-1548789916

Other books by Polly Fielding

Single Serving Vegetarian Recipes To Soothe Arthritis

Single Serving Recipes To Soothe Arthritis

Vegetarian Recipes For One To Lower Blood Pressure

The 5:2 Diet Made eZy

The 5:2 Vegetarian Diet Made eZy

Mindfulness For The 5:2 Diet

Moments of Mindfulness

Time for Mindfulness

Nurturing Compassion

A Veritable Smorgasbord

Missing Factor

Going In Seine

Breaking The Silence

Letting Go (a trilogy comprising the three books below)

And This Is My Adopted Daughter

A Mind To Be Free

Crossing The Borderline

www.pollyfielding.com

To John and Michael, with love

CONTENTS

Acknowledgement

Grateful thanks to Jayne Richardson, diabetes nurse, for her helpful advice on the contents of this book

Introduction

It came as a shock when my sister told me, several months ago, that she had recently been diagnosed with diabetes type 2. Although somewhat overweight, she is a vegetarian and I always got the impression that she ate pretty healthily.

However, she confided to me that as a 'foodie', she had paid little attention to her diet for many years and led too busy a life running her little craft shop to even think about doing any exercise.

Yet, despite being willing to seriously review her diet and lifestyle in the light of her diagnosis, she was finding it really difficult trying to figure out how radical any changes should be. She was getting confused about the fair amount of seemingly conflicting advice about what to do if you have diabetes.

I decided that I would tackle the subject myself, develop an understanding of diabetes and find out what would be most helpful on a day- to- day basis to live healthily with it. Then I would devise suitable recipes for someone cooking just for themselves, like my sister.

And since I myself would prefer simple, straightforward answers to the kinds of questions my sister asked, I have written the first part of this book in question and answer form.

I discovered that not only is it possible to live well with diabetes but that the recommended diet is not that different from the sort we should all be eating regularly, whether we have diabetes or not. Contrary to some people's expectations, it does not mean sticking to a boring, bland diet. In compiling these recipes I have paid particular attention to the balance of carbohydrates, and the nutritional content of meals (protein, fat, sodium, fibre and calories) whilst also ensuring that they are varied, colourful and enjoyable.

It all comes down to a combination of moderation in your eating following sensible guidelines (including any that are specifically given to you by your GP and diabetes nurse) and increasing the amount you exercise, such as going for a daily brisk twenty minute walk. These measures will enable you to give yourself the best chance possible to keep well and get the most out of life.

Understanding Diabetes

What is diabetes?

Diabetes, in simple terms, is a condition where too much sugar remains in your blood (sometimes it's called 'sweet blood'). This sugar, also known as 'glucose', is not able to enter the cells of your body effectively to be used as fuel to keep you healthy.

There are two main types of diabetes: type 1 and type 2.

In the case of type 1, no insulin is produced by an organ in the body called the pancreas and, since insulin is responsible for controlling glucose, it builds up in the bloodstream, unable to get used.

In type 2 diabetes, however, your body can still produce insulin but either it's insufficient for its requirements or it's unable to be used properly.

Why did I develop this condition?

Although there is a genetic component to both kinds, the cause of type 1 diabetes is unrelated to diet and lifestyle whereas the reason for the occurrence of type 2 diabetes is often significantly linked to both. The rising levels of diabetes type 2 are increasing globally in line with mounting levels of obesity. This book is primarily aimed at the second group, which is the most common.

What are the implications of having diabetes?

Left untreated, diabetes would be very dangerous to someone's health resulting in potentially serious diseases such as those affecting the heart, kidneys, skin, eyes, feet, blood vessels...

How is it treated?

Although there is currently no cure once you have this condition, with sensible changes to diet, lifestyle - and, if necessary, the addition of medication - it can be successfully controlled so that you can live a normal, healthy life.

The aim of any treatment is to keep your blood sugar under control, so your doctor or diabetes nurse will ensure that you regularly get your blood tested (at least annually) to determine your ongoing blood glucose levels. Your weight, blood pressure and cholesterol levels will also be monitored.

Type 1 diabetics are taught how to inject themselves with insulin, carry out daily blood sugar checks and manage their diet with regular healthy, balanced meals and snacks.

If you are a type 2 diabetic you can usually manage with

medication in tablet form in addition to losing weight if you need to (particularly around your waist), increasing the amount of exercise you take, cutting down on your intake of alcohol, not smoking and making important changes to your diet. This last point can be very confusing for someone with diabetes and needs more explanation.

Does having diabetes mean that I can never have anything containing sugar?

Since any changes to your diet need to be maintained over your lifetime, they must be realistic. Eating should be a pleasurable activity for anyone, including diabetics, so the answer to this question is not black and white. Avoiding sugar (which is high in calories anyway), whenever you can, makes good sense - don't add it to drinks or cereals and, generally speaking, reserve any sugary food for the occasional treat.

If you have a 'sweet tooth' there are plenty of viable alternatives to sugar - many supermarkets now stock sugar-free jams, chocolate and biscuits... And there are non-chemical sweeteners that can be safely added to food such as plant-based stevia.

A high intake of sugar, particularly if it's not part of a meal, can cause a spike in your blood glucose which can make you suddenly feel quite unwell. Conversely, if you do not eat regular, properly balanced meals your blood glucose level could drop too low and result in feeling ill.

So what is meant by a 'balanced' diet?

Basically, the recommended balanced diet for someone with diabetes is no different from the kind of healthy eating style everyone should be following. This means eating foods that are low in salt, sugar and saturated fat but high in starch, fibre, vegetables and fruit.

I have been advised to make sure that I choose foods that have a low glycaemic index to include in my meals. What does this mean?

The glycaemic Index (GI) on a scale of 0 - 100 is the measure of the extent to which carbohydrates in food increase your blood sugar level. Foods such beans, oats, wholegrains, lentils, pasta, most vegetables and sweet fruits have a low GI. The lower the GI, the less you will have fluctuations in your blood sugar after you have eaten.

Since sweet potatoes have a slightly lower GI than white potatoes - the starch in them is converted into blood glucose more slowly - I have chosen to include them in some of my recipes. As well as being rich in healthy fibre, they are also high in nutrients such as vitamin A and potassium.

Breakfasts

Index of Breakfasts

Roasted Tomatoes on Toast

Ingredients

3 medium tomatoes, halved

sprinkle of ground black pepper

½ tsp freshly chopped chives

2 tsp dried wholemeal breadcrumbs

1 tsp low fat cheddar cheese, finely grated

1 slice wholemeal bread

Method

- Preheat oven to 190°C
- Place tomatoes (cut side up) on a baking sheet
- Sprinkle with pepper & chives
- Roast for approx. 10 minutes
- Sprinkle breadcrumbs & cheese over them
- Roast for a further 5 minutes
- Meanwhile, toast bread in toaster
- Put toast on a plate & top with the tomatoes
- Serve & enjoy!

Boiled Egg with Asparagus

Ingredients

1 large egg
olive oil spray
12g dried breadcrumbs
pinch of chilli powder
pinch of paprika
4 asparagus spears
1 slice wholemeal bread
1 tsp olive oil spread

Method

- Fry the breadcrumbs gently in 4 sprays of hot oil until golden blown
- Mix in the chilli, paprika & place to one side
- Place the asparagus in a saucepan of boiling water & cook until tender (about 5 minutes)
- While the asparagus is cooking, cook the egg in a pan of boiling water for approximately 5 minutes
- Meanwhile toast bread & cover with spread
- Put the egg in an egg cup in the middle of a plate and arrange the drained asparagus around it
- Sprinkle the crumbs over the asparagus
- Arrange toast cut in half either side of plate
- It's ready to eat!

Apricot & Banana Bagel

Ingredients

1 wholemeal bagel

10g dried apricots, chopped

20g low-fat soft cheese

1 small banana, sliced

Method

- Preheat grill
- Cut bagel in half & toast, cut sides up
- Meanwhile, combine low-fat soft cheese & chopped apricots
- Spread mixture equally onto toasted bagel halves
- Top with banana slices
- Serve
- Bon appétit!

Pineapple and Cottage Cheese Toastie

Ingredients

1 slice wholemeal bread

28g cottage cheese

1 teaspoon cinnamon

1 slice pineapple

Method

- Preheat the grill to a medium heat
- Toast the bread lightly on both sides
- Spread the cottage cheese evenly over the toast
- Sprinkle with the cinnamon
- Place the pineapple on top
- Put the toastie under the grill
- Grill until the cheese begins to brown
- Serve with pride!

Mediterranean Oaty Breakfast

Ingredients

4 large sun-dried tomato halves, not oil-packed,
thinly sliced
240ml vegetable stock
ground black pepper to taste
1 tbsp fresh chives, very finely chopped
112g oats
3 tbsp natural, fat-free Greek yoghurt
1 tbsp soft goat cheese, crumbled
1 tbsp fresh basil, finely chopped

Method

- Place sun-dried tomatoes with the stock in a small saucepan, season with pepper & bring to the boil over a medium high heat
- Add in chives & oats
- Stir continuously for approx 5 minutes until oats are cooked
- Remove from heat & gently stir in the yogurt
- Spoon into serving bowl
- Sprinkle the cheese & basil onto the mixture
- Eat slowly & mindfully

Poached Egg on Bed of Avocado

Ingredients

1 slice of wholemeal bread

small ripe avocado

1 free-range egg

extra virgin olive oil

Method

- Lightly toast the bread
- Meanwhile, peel and slice avocado
- Drizzle a little oil onto the toast
- Place avocado slices on the toast
- Poach the egg
- Place egg on top of avocado
- Relish each mouthful

Green Smoothie

Ingredients

100ml unsweetened jasmine green tea (made with 1 tea bag)

½ tsp grated fresh ginger root

¼ cucumber, chopped

112g frozen mango cubes

30g fresh baby spinach

1 tbsp packed fresh mint leaves

1 tsp fresh lime juice

½ tbsp lemon juice

Method

- Put all above ingredients into a blender
- Whizz on high setting until completely smooth
- Pour into a large glass
- Savour each sip

Spicy Toastie

Ingredients

1 slice of wholemeal bread
1 tsp all natural peanut butter
1 tbsp natural fat-free yoghurt
1 small banana, sliced
pinch of cinnamon
pinch of mixed spice
pinch of ground ginger

Method

- Mix the peanut butter and yoghurt thoroughly in a bowl
- Toast the bread
- Spread the mixture on the toast & place slices of banana on top
- Season with cinnamon, mixed spice & ginger
- Serve & enjoy!

Creamy Nutty Breakfast

Ingredients

165g Greek yoghurt

30g mixed nuts

1 tbsp wheat bran

10g rolled oats

10g chia seeds

1 kiwi fruit, peeled & sliced

Method

- Spoon yoghurt into a cereal bowl
- Add nuts, wheat bran, oats & chia seeds
- Arrange kiwi slices over
- Your breakfast is ready!

Polenta Surprise

Ingredients

75ml semi-skimmed milk

110ml water

75g dry polenta

75ml low fat single cream

75g blueberries

stevia, to taste

Method

- Pour milk & water into a small saucepan & bring to the boil
- Turn heat down & stir in polenta
- Keep stirring until the liquid is absorbed
- Scoop into a serving bowl
- Add stevia to taste
- Stir in cream
- Top with blueberries
- Enjoy!

Cheesy Mushrooms on Toast

Ingredients

1 slice wholemeal bread

1½ tbsp light cream cheese

1 tsp olive oil

100g small flat mushrooms, sliced

1tbsp semi-skimmed milk

¼ tsp wholegrain mustard

1 tbsp chives, chopped

Method

- Toast bread
- Spread with ½ of the cheese
- Heat oil in a non-stick frying pan & stir in mushrooms & cook until softened
- Stir in milk, mustard & rest of the cheese until mushrooms are well coated
- Scoop onto toast
- Sprinkle chives over & serve yourself

Mushroom with Spinach Frittata

Ingredients

1-calorie olive oil spray

80 g fresh mushrooms, chopped

10g baby spinach leaves, stems

1 large egg

1 tbsp feta cheese

freshly ground black pepper to taste

Method

- Use 4 sprays of oil in small non-stick frying pan
- Heat on medium heat
- Sauté mushrooms for 3 minutes
- Add spinach leaves & cook for approx 30 seconds until spinach wilts
- Whisk egg in small bowl with pepper
- Pour egg mixture over mushrooms and spinach
- Allow egg to set over medium-high heat, lifting edges to let any uncooked egg flow to sides.
- When frittata is almost set, sprinkle the feta cheese over it
- Place under medium grill until cheese is melted & lightly browned (approx 3 minutes)
- Serve & eat while hot

Blueberry Porridge

Ingredients

25g blueberries
75ml apple juice
25g porridge oats
300ml water

Method

- Put blueberries in a small saucepan
- Pour in the apple juice
- Bring to the boil on a medium-high heat, stir then simmer for 5 minutes
- Remove from heat & allow to cool for approx 10 minutes
- Scoop into blender & blend until puréed
- Tip oats into a small saucepan & cover with the water
- Cook for 3–4 minutes over gentle heat, stirring occasionally
- Put the porridge into a bowl & stir in the blueberry purée
- Savour each delicious mouthful

Chia Delight

Ingredients

50ml water

100ml unsweetened almond milk

50g quinoa

25g chia seeds

1 tsp raw cocoa powder

stevia to taste

30g blueberries

Method

- Pour water & milk into a saucepan
- Add quinoa
- Heat until it boils
- Reduce heat & simmer for 15 minutes
- Transfer to a serving bowl
- Mix in the chia seeds, cocoa & stevia
- Top with blueberries
- Yummy!

Tasty Burrito

Ingredients

1 tbsp semi-skimmed milk

2 small eggs

1 small tomato, finely chopped

½ green pepper, deseeded & chopped finely

½ spring onion, finely chopped

½ tsp vegetable oil

10g reduced-fat hard cheese, grated

sprinkle of ground black pepper

1 soft wholewheat flour tortilla

Method

- Preheat the grill
- Whisk milk & eggs in small bowl
- In a different bowl, mix tomato, spring onions, chopped pepper & ground pepper
- Put vegetable oil into a non-stick frying pan & heat gently
- Add beaten egg mixture
- Cook over medium heat briefly until base is set
- Pour tomato mixture onto the egg
- Sprinkle cheese over
- Grill to set the egg and melt the cheese

- Slide omelette onto the tortilla
- Leave a while to cool
- Roll up the tortilla
- Use a sharp knife to slice in half before serving

Muesli & Apple Smoothie

Ingredients

2 tbsp sugar-free muesli

1 apple, peeled, cored and chopped

150ml skimmed milk

150g carton low-fat natural yogurt

Method

- Put all the above ingredients into a blender
- Blend until a smooth consistency is achieved
- Transfer to an attractive bowl & breakfast in style

Weekend Fruity Chia Breakfast

Ingredients

240ml almond milk
60ml canned coconut milk
2 tbsp chia seeds
¼ inch knob fresh ginger, minced
½ teaspoon vanilla extract
1 small mango, peeled, de-stoned & diced
small sprinkle of shredded, unsweetened coconut
1 tsp raspberries
slice of fresh lime
small sprig fresh mint

Method

- Pour almond & coconut milk into serving bowl
- Stir in chia seeds ginger, vanilla & soak until it jellifies (approx 1 hour), stirring occasionally
- Top with diced mango
- Sprinkle coconut over
- Top with raspberries
- Garnish with lime slice & mint
- Looks good & taste heavenly!

Total Toasty Beany Breakfast

Ingredients

1 spring onion, chopped finely

¼ red pepper, deseeded & chopped finely

1 tbsp water

¼ can baked beans (reduced salt & sugar)

4 cherry tomatoes, halved

40g mushrooms, sliced

1 medium slice wholemeal bread

1 tsp low fat spread

freshly ground black pepper

Method

- Put chopped spring onion & pepper into a large saucepan with the water. Cook over gentle heat for 2 minutes or until the water has evaporated
- Add the beans, tomatoes & mushrooms and heat gently for approx 5 minutes, stirring frequently, until the mixture is thoroughly heated
- Meanwhile, toast the slice of bread
- Evenly cover the toast with the spread
- Spoon beany mixture onto the toast
- Sprinkle with black pepper to taste
- Serve while still hot

Poached Egg with Mushrooms

Ingredients

1 slice wholemeal bread

1 small egg

1 drop of vinegar

56g button mushrooms, wiped clean with a damp paper towel

1-cal vegetable oil spray

Method

- Boil a half-filled medium saucepan of water
- Use 4 sprays of 1-cal oil to coat a small non-stick frying pan & heat gently
- Break egg into a cup & add a drop of vinegar which will help the egg to keep its shape during cooking
- Stir the boiling water vigorously to make it swirl and drop egg into the middle
- On a low heat, cook for approx. 3 minutes
- Toast the bread
- Meanwhile, fry mushrooms on medium heat, keeping them moving in the pan until golden (around 3 minutes)
- Using a slotted spoon, remove egg from the water & drain on piece of kitchen towel

- Place egg in centre of toast, surround with the mushrooms
- Serve immediately

Nutty Muesli

Ingredients

30g oats

tip of tsp stevia (optional)

50ml skimmed milk

50ml water

1 apple, grated (no need to peel)

1 tbsp fat-free live yogurt

2 strawberries, chopped

10g chopped unsalted pistachio nuts

pinch of cinnamon

Method

- If using stevia to sweeten, mix into oats in a bowl
- Add milk & water & soak for 45 minutes or - even better - leave overnight in the fridge
- Stir grated apple into oats
- Spoon on the yogurt
- Top with strawberries & nuts
- Sprinkle with cinnamon
- Eat & enjoy every mouthful!

Fruity Couscous

Ingredients

120ml skimmed milk

56g couscous

28g blueberries

28g seedless grapes

stevia to taste (optional)

Method

- Heat milk in microwave until hot (approx 40 seconds or less, depending on your microwave)
- Add couscous to milk & allow to stand for 5 minutes
- Stir in grapes & blueberries
- Add stevia to taste if desired
- Serve & enjoy

Strawberry Delight

Ingredients

1 small pot natural fat-free yoghurt

1 heaped tbsp strawberries, chopped

2 sugar-free digestive biscuits, crushed

Method

- Scoop yoghurt into serving bowl
- Stir strawberries into yoghurt
- Top with crushed biscuits and serve

Scrambled Egg with a Difference

Ingredients

1 large egg

1 tbsp semi-skimmed milk

small sprinkle garlic powder

ground black pepper

1 tbsp salsa

1 tbsp reduced fat cheese

1 slice wholemeal bread, toasted & lightly covered
with a vegetable-based spread

Method

- Crack the egg into a microwave-safe bowl
- Add milk
- Sprinkle in the garlic powder & ground pepper, to taste
- Whisk mixture
- Cook mixture in microwave until egg is cooked through, for about 1 minute (stirring briskly with fork after 40 seconds then cooking for further 20)
- Meanwhile toast bread & butter it
- Transfer scrambled egg to toast
- Top with the salsa
- Sprinkle cheese over & serve

Apple and Walnut Porridge

Ingredients

30g porridge oats

10g sultanas

10g chopped walnuts

100ml unsweetened apple juice

Method

- Mix all ingredients well in a microwaveable bowl
- Microwave for 1½ minutes (based on 700W – adjust time accordingly)
- Stir & serve

Creamy Strawberry & Almond Crunch

Ingredients

30g bran flakes

100ml fat free natural yoghurt

75g chopped almonds

5 strawberries, chopped

Method

- Put half the bran flakes into a cereal bowl
- Spoon half the yoghurt over the bran
- Sprinkle on half the almonds & half the strawberries
- Cover with the remainder of the bran
- Spoon the rest of the yoghurt over
- Sprinkle on the remaining almonds & strawberries
- Savour each delicious mouthful!

Lunches

Index of Lunches

Quick Spiced Sweet Potato Lunch

Ingredients

1 large sweet potato

4 tbsp natural, fat-free yoghurt

cinnamon to taste

lettuce for side salad

Method

- Use a fork to prick sweet potato skin in several places
- Wrap in kitchen paper and microwave on highest setting for approx 6 minutes (until soft) turning once
- Cut sweet potato in half, lengthwise
- Spoon yoghurt onto potato
- Sprinkle with cinnamon
- Serve with lettuce

Asparagus Omelette

Ingredients

1-cal olive oil spray
2 eggs
1 tsp fresh herbs, finely chopped
ground black pepper, to taste
5 asparagus tips
4 cherry tomatoes, halved
sprig of parsley

Method

- Cook asparagus in a few inches of boiling water in a covered saucepan for approx. 8 minutes (until tips are tender)
- Drain, return to pan & cover to keep warm
- Coat an omelette pan with 4 sprays of 1-cal olive oil & heat gently over medium heat
- Whisk egg
- Add herbs, pepper to taste
- Pour mixture into pan and spread evenly
- When set, & golden on the underside, arrange asparagus on one side & fold omelette in half
- Slide onto warmed plate
- Serve garnished with parsley & decorated with tomatoes

Butterbean Dip with Vegetable Batons

Ingredients

100g tinned butterbeans, drained

1 spring onion, finely chopped

20g cucumber, finely diced

2 tsp low-fat, natural yogurt

1 small clove garlic, crushed

1 tsp extra-virgin olive oil

1 tsp zest of lemon

2 tsp lemon juice

sprig of fresh mint, chopped

pinch of pepper

pinch of paprika

small stick of celery, cut into batons

small carrot, cut into batons

small yellow pepper, cut into batons

Method

- Mash beans with a fork until smooth
- Stir in spring onions, cucumber, yogurt, garlic, olive oil, lemon, mint and pepper
- Sprinkle with paprika
- Serve with vegetable batons, relishing each tasty mouthful

Mediterranean Sandwich

Ingredients

1 round of multigrain sandwich thins

2 tsp olive oil

1 tsp fresh rosemary

1 egg

112g baby spinach leaves

1 small tomato, sliced thinly

1 tbsp reduced-fat feta cheese

ground black pepper, to taste

Method

- Preheat oven to 190°C
- Separate sandwich thins
- Brush cut sides with 1 tsp of olive oil (i.e. ½ tsp each)
- Put onto baking sheet
- Bake in oven for approx. 5 minutes (until edges are lightly browned)
- Meanwhile, heat the remaining tsp olive oil with rosemary in a frying pan over medium-high heat
- Break egg into the frying pan
- Cook until white is set but yolk is still runny
- Break yolk with spatula & turn egg over to cook, for a few seconds, on other side

- Remove from heat
- Put bottom half of toasted sandwich thins on a serving plates
- Top with spinach
- Add tomato slices, egg, & cheese
- Sprinkle with pepper, to taste
- Cover with the remaining sandwich thin & enjoy each bite!

Veggie Risotto

Ingredients

1 tbsp olive oil

4 sage leaves, shredded

2 leeks, sliced

85g risotto rice

200ml hot vegetable stock

small glass white wine

2 large mushrooms

3 tbsp reduced fat cheese, grated

ground black pepper

Method

- Heat oil in small non-stick frying pan
- Fry leeks & sage for approx. 2 minutes (until the leeks soften)
- Add rice, stir continuously, cooking for 1 min
- Pour in stock & wine & bring to the boil
- Turn heat down to low, cover pan & simmer for approx. 10 minutes (until rice is cooked)
- Meanwhile, grill mushrooms
- Remove rice from heat, stir in cheese & add ground pepper.
- Transfer risotto to a plate

- Top with grilled mushrooms
- Serve with a self-satisfied smile!

Cheesy Spiced Omelette

Ingredients

4 sprigs of fresh coriander, finely chopped
1 spring onion, finely chopped
pinch of dried chilli flakes
1 tbsp olive oil
2 large eggs
25g reduced fat cheddar cheese, grated
ground black pepper to taste

Method

- Chop coriander & spring onion finely
- Whisk eggs, adding pepper to taste
- In a small frying pan heat the oil
- Add coriander & onion to frying pan, sprinkle on the chilli flakes & stir until slightly softened
- Pour in eggs, stirring until almost set
- Sprinkle the cheese over and cook for approx. 1 minute (until omelette is set & cheese has melted)
- Use a spatula to fold the omelette over in half
- Slide carefully onto a plate
- Consume slowly, savouring each mouthful

Feta Wrap

Ingredients

1 x 10-inch whole-wheat tortilla

42g feta cheese, crumbled

2 black olives, sliced

¼ small yellow squash, sliced

¼ cucumber, diced

4 cherry tomatoes, halved

1 small red onion, thinly sliced

2 tsp balsamic vinegar

small clove garlic, minced

2 tsp chopped fresh parsley

1 tsp olive oil

ground black pepper

Method

- In a bowl mix all the ingredients together (except for the tortilla)
- Allow to stand for 15 minutes, stirring occasionally
- Drain off any liquid & place mixture on tortilla
- Fold bottom of wrap over lower part of filling
- Roll up the tortilla
- It's a wrap!

Avocado & Strawberry Lunch

Ingredients

2 tsp lemon juice

½ ripe avocado, peeled & chopped

60g chopped strawberries

1 tsp extra virgin olive oil

2 tsp raspberry vinegar

½ tsp honey

freshly ground black pepper, to taste

112g watercress

2 tsp toasted pine nuts

Method

- Mix lemon juice with avocado in a bowl
- Put in strawberries, oil, vinegar, honey, pepper & stir thoroughly
- Place a bed of watercress on a plate
- Transfer avocado & berry mixture onto the watercress
- Sprinkle with pine nuts
- Enjoy!

Lime & Chili Coated Corn on the Cob

Ingredients

1 large corn on the cob
juice of ½ lime
½ tsp lime zest
2 tsp olive oil margarine
¼ tsp chilli powder
mixed salad of your choice

Method

- Preheat grill to medium
- Mix lime juice, lime zest, margarine & chilli powder in a small bowl
- Spread mixture evenly over the cob
- Grill for approx. 20 minutes, turning frequently
- Serve on an attractive plate with your salad
- Looks attractive & tastes delicious!

Edamame Bean Salad

Ingredients

Salad:

50g edamame beans
handful of mixed salad leaves
2 spring onions, finely sliced
6 slices of cucumber
1 large tomato, sliced
half a punnet of cress

Tahini dressing :

1 tbsp fat-free natural yogurt
1 tsp tahini (sesame paste)

Garnish:

½ tsp sesame seeds
1 lemon wedge
generous pinch of black pepper

Method

- Put the edamame beans, salad leaves & spring onions into a bowl
- Add cucumber, tomato & cress
- In another bowl, mix together the yogurt & tahini
- Stir this dressing into the bowl of salad
- Transfer to a serving plate
- Sprinkle with sesame seeds & black pepper
- Serve with the wedge of lemon

Hot Vegetable & Pesto Slice

Ingredients

56g courgette slices

56g yellow squash slices

56g red pepper slices

1 tbsp reduced-fat balsamic vinaigrette dressing

½ garlic clove, minced

1-cal olive oil cooking spray

2 tsp pesto

1 slice wholemeal bread

1 tbsp reduced-fat cheddar cheese, shredded

Method

- Preheat grill to medium
- Put courgette, squash & pepper slices into a large bowl
- Stir in balsamic dressing & garlic thoroughly
- Spray grill pan with oil
- Place vegetables in grill pan, spray lightly with oil and cook for approx. 4 minutes on each side (until tender)
- Meanwhile, spread pesto onto bread slice
- Remove vegetables from heat, put briefly to one side & turn grill to high

- Line a baking tin with foil
- Top pesto bread slice evenly with the cooked vegetables & sprinkle the cheese over
- Place on baking tin & grill until cheeses melts, around 2-3 minutes
- Transfer to a serving plate & eat while hot

Mixed Vegetable Frittata

Ingredients

1 tsp olive oil

1 small tomato, chopped

1 small green pepper, deseeded, & chopped

1 large mushroom, roughly chopped

½ courgette, finely chopped

2 eggs

1 tbsp semi-skimmed milk

1 slice wholemeal bread

 pinch of ground black pepper

Method

- Preheat grill
- In a non-stick frying pan, heat the oil
- Spread tomato, pepper, mushroom & courgette out in the frying pan & cook gently for 3-4 minutes, (until soft) stirring frequently
- Whisk eggs & milk & pour evenly over vegetables
- Cook on medium heat for 4-5 minutes to set base of frittata
- Use a spatula to transfer the frittata to a foil-lined grill pan
- Grill for 2-3 minutes until surface is cooked

- Toast the bread
- Put the frittata onto a serving plate

Vegetable Soup with Beans

Ingredients

1 teaspoons olive oil

½ small stick celery, finely chopped

1 small onion, finely sliced

140g chopped spinach

1 small can salt-free chopped tomatoes, undrained

150ml vegetable stock

1 tbsp fresh parsley

½ tsp dried marjoram

Small pinch cayenne pepper

Small sprinkle ground nutmeg

75g canned butter beans, drained

crispbreads

Method

- Coat a medium, non-stick frying pan with oil & heat gently
- Add celery & onions & cook for 4 - 5 minutes, or until celery is tender, stirring occasionally.
- Add spinach & stir well
- Cook for 2 - 3 minutes, stirring frequently, (until any liquid evaporates) & mixture comes away easily from sides of pan

- Stir in the rest of the ingredients apart from the butter beans
- Cover & bring to the boil on medium high heat
- Turn down heat & simmer, still covered, for approx. 10 minutes (until vegetables are tender)
- Add in the beans, leave pan uncovered & cook on medium heat for 1 minute (until the beans are piping hot)
- Scoop into serving bowl & enjoy with a couple of crispbreads

Green Veggie Soup

Ingredients

3 sticks celery, chopped

¼ leek, sliced

50g spinach

300ml vegetable stock

1-cal olive oil spray

½ tablespoon fat-free yoghurt

Method

- Use 5 sprays of olive oil to coat a frying pan
- Fry the leek & celery on a gentle heat for approximately 5 minutes, (until the leeks are soft)
- Add stock & cook for 25 minutes on a low heat
- Mix in the spinach & continue to cook for 5 minutes
- Pour the mixture into a blender & liquidize
- Swirl in the yoghurt & serve

Simple Yogurt & Vegetable Dip

Ingredients

½ stick celery

1 small carrot

2 small florets broccoli

½ red pepper, deseeded

½ tsp minced fresh dill

Small squeeze fresh lemon juice

freshly ground black pepper to taste

1 small pot natural, fat-free yogurt

Method

- Cut celery & pepper into batons
- Peel carrot & slice into batons
- Spoon yoghurt into small bowl
- Stir in dill & ground pepper
- Squeeze in lemon juice & stir
- Place bowl in centre of a large plate
- Arrange celery, pepper & carrot batons with broccoli around bowl
- It's ready!

Goat's Cheese with a Light Crunchy Salad

Ingredients

30g goat's cheese

1 tomato, finely chopped

Small sprig fresh mint, chopped

10g fresh coriander, roughly chopped

juice and finely grated zest of ¼ lemon

1 tsp extra virgin olive oil

pinch pepper

60g grated carrot

½ small red onion, finely diced

40g cucumber, finely diced

Method

- Put all ingredients, except goat's cheese, into a medium-sized bowl
- Mix thoroughly together
- Tip onto attractive serving plate
- Add goat's cheese
- Enjoy mindfully!

Chive & Courgette Omelette

Ingredients

2 small eggs

1 courgette, finely diced

1 teaspoon chives, chopped

1-cal spray olive oil

ground black pepper

Method

- Whisk the eggs thoroughly
- Add the courgette and chives
- Season pepper
- Spray a frying pan with olive oil and heat on a medium setting
- Pour in the egg mixture
- Cook until firm on one side then flip over and cook until the base is golden brown
- Serve immediately

Bulgur Wheat with Roasted Pepper & Tomato

Ingredients

35g bulgur wheat

1 small red pepper, chopped

150g cherry tomatoes

2 tsp balsamic vinegar

freshly ground black pepper

2 tsp olive oil

2 tsp fresh basil, chopped

sprig of parsley

Method

- Preheat oven to 220°C
- Put bulgur wheat into a bowl & pour on boiling water until just covered
- Soak for 30 minutes, then drain off any excess liquid
- Meanwhile put red pepper & tomatoes onto a baking sheet & roast for 10 - 15 minutes (until soft)
- Mix vinegar, oil & basil into bulgur wheat
- Sprinkle with black pepper
- Garnish with parsley sprig
- Munch mindfully

A Quick Lunch

Ingredients

5 whole wheat crackers
1 tsp all natural peanut butter
1 hard-boiled egg, sliced
1 apple
1 small carrot, peeled

Method

- Peel carrot & cut into sticks
- Cut apple into quarters
- Arrange carrot sticks, apple quarters & egg slices alternately round edge of a serving plate
- Spread peanut butter onto crackers & place them in the centre of the plate
- Enjoy each bite

Vegetable Chilli

Ingredients

½ clove garlic, crushed

½ red chilli, chopped

¼ teaspoon ground cumin

65g mushrooms, quartered

100g canned kidney beans

100g canned chopped tomatoes

40g green beans, trimmed and sliced

50ml water

1 teaspoon low-fat crème fraîche

piece of crusty bread

1-cal olive oil spray

Method

- Spray a frying pan four times with the olive oil and heat
- Put in garlic & chilli & fry for 2 minutes
- Add mushrooms & cumin & cook for a further 3 minutes
- Pour in tomatoes, kidney beans & water
- Simmer for 10 minutes, stirring occasionally
- Mix in the green beans & cook for five more minutes until sauce thickens & beans are soft

- Pour into serving bowl, top with crème fraîche & enjoy with crusty bread

Black Bean Salad

Ingredients

Dressing:

1 small pot natural, fat free, yogurt
1 small handful packed fresh coriander
½ ripe avocado, chopped
2 spring onions, finely chopped
1 small clove garlic, quartered
1 tablespoon lime juice
small pinch of stevia

Salad:

2 large handfuls mixed greens
1 tomato, chopped
112g tinned black beans, rinsed
112g frozen sweetcorn, thawed

Method

- Put yogurt, coriander, avocado, spring onions, garlic, lime juice & stevia into a blender & whisk until smooth

- Place greens in a salad bowl
- Mix in 2 tbsp of the dressing
- Store remaining dressing in a small covered container in fridge for another day
- Add black beans, tomato & sweetcorn to salad greens
- Your lunch is ready

Vegetable Broth

Ingredients

2 tsp olive oil

1 small onion, chopped

1 tsp chopped rosemary

½ small garlic clove, chopped

1 small carrot, chopped

215ml vegetable stock

100g can chickpeas, drained

25g green beans, chopped

Method

- Heat the oil in a small pan over a medium heat.
- Add onion, rosemary and garlic and fry for 2 minutes
- Add carrots and pour in stock
- Simmer for 10 minutes before mixing in the chickpeas
- Stir in the beans and simmer for a further 3 minutes
- Serve and enjoy

Vegetable Stir Fry

Ingredients

1-cal olive oil spray

4 spring onions, thinly sliced

1 tablespoon root ginger, chopped finely

1 clove garlic, chopped

½ small yellow pepper, sliced thinly

½ small red pepper, sliced thinly

1 leaf choi sum., shredded

56g bean sprouts

56g sugar snaps peas

1 tablespoon sesame oil

2 tablespoons soy sauce

Method

- Coat a wok well with olive oil spray (6 sprays)
- Fry the onions, ginger, garlic & peppers gently until soft (about 3 minutes)
- Add the choi sum, bean sprouts & peas, together with the soy sauce and sesame oil
- Stir fry for a further 2 minutes before serving

Tofu, Hazelnut & Chestnut Mushroom Pâté with Toast

Ingredients

1 tsp olive oil

¼ small red onion, finely sliced

40g chestnut mushrooms, sliced

1 tsp brandy

25g roasted hazelnuts

1 slice wholemeal bread

64g smoked tofu, chopped

1 tsp tamari

¼ tsp fresh thyme

freshly ground black pepper

Method

- Heat oil in a frying pan & fry onion slices until golden brown
- Mix in the mushrooms & continue frying for approx 3 minutes (until softened & an even brown)
- Meanwhile toast bread, cut in half & arrange either side of a serving plate
- Add brandy to the mushrooms & onions & remove from heat
- Grind roasted hazelnuts in a blender

- Add tofu, tamari, onions, mushrooms & thyme & blend until smooth; if necessary adding a splash of water to achieve smooth, firm consistency
- Season with pepper, transfer to the serving plate to enjoy with the toast

Mushroom Burger

Ingredients

Marinade (allow approx. 2 hours for this)

½ tbsp olive oil

2 tbsp low sodium soy sauce

1 large clove garlic, crushed

2 tbsp balsamic vinegar

Burger

2 x 10cm portobello mushroom caps

15cm long thin crusty baguette

2 thin slices of onion

3 slices of tomato

2 leaves of romaine lettuce

mustard or relish, to taste

Method

- Put oil, soy sauce, garlic & vinegar into a zip-topped sandwich bag
- Add in the mushrooms & gently shake until mushrooms are coated

- Leave to marinate for approx. 2 hours (at room temperature), occasionally shaking gently
- Preheat oven to 260°C
- Remove mushrooms & discard bag & remaining marinade
- Put mushrooms on a baking tray & roast for 4 minutes
- Turn mushrooms over & cook for a further 2 minutes
- Remove mushrooms from heat
- Cut baguette into half
- Put mushrooms on one half, top with onion, tomato slices, lettuce & mustard or relish
- Cover with the other half of the baguette & tuck in!

Polly Fielding

Dinners

Index of Dinners

Herby Mushroom Risotto

Ingredients

1 tsp olive oil

100g chestnut mushrooms, sliced

25g quinoa

250ml hot vegetable stock

45g brown risotto rice

a few thyme leaves

56g reduced fat cheddar cheese, grated

20g rocket

Method

- Heat oil in a medium saucepan,
- Add the mushrooms & sauté for 2 mins
- Stir quinoa into the pan
- Add one ladle of vegetable stock & stir until absorbed.
- Stir in rice & add another ladle of the stock & stir until it's absorbed
- Repeat this process until all the stock is used up & rice & quinoa are cooked
- Stir thyme leaves into the mixture
- Spoon onto a plate
- Sprinkle grated cheese over it & serve with the rocket

Baked Smoked Tofu with Couscous

Ingredients

1 tsp olive oil

150g smoked tofu

100g couscous

250ml vegetable stock

1 small red pepper, finely chopped

1 onion, finely chopped

1 tbsp fresh parsley, chopped

1 tbsp pesto sauce

juice & zest of 1 lemon

freshly ground black pepper

Method

- Preheat oven to 200°C
- Heat oil in a non-stick frying pan
- Fry tofu for 2 minutes each side until golden brown
- Put couscous into an ovenproof dish
- Stir in stock, red pepper, onion, parsley, lemon juice & zest
- Pour onto the couscous & stir
- Place the tofu on top of the couscous,
- Spoon on the pesto & season with pepper

- Cover with foil & bake for 20 minutes
- Fluff up couscous with a fork before serving
- Serve with a smile!

Soya Mince Loaf with Sweet Potato & Peas

Ingredients

1 tbsp oil

100g onion, chopped finely

50g red pepper, deseeded & chopped

1 tsp garlic, chopped finely

15g wholemeal breadcrumbs

1 vegetable stock cube

1 medium egg

1 tsp tomato purée

50g soya mince

½ tsp ground fennel seeds

25ml semi-skimmed milk

25g pine nuts

50g sun-dried tomatoes, drained of oil & chopped

½ tsp dried rosemary

½ tsp dried oregano

1 medium sweet potato, cut into quarters & boiled

2 tbsp peas

sprig of parsley to garnish

Method

- Preheat the oven to 190°C

- Meanwhile, heat oil on low heat
- Add the onions, red pepper & garlic & cook, stirring frequently for approx 8 min
- Add the tomato purée and cook, stirring regularly for 2 min, then remove from the heat and allow to cool
- Crumble stock cube into breadcrumbs & mix well
- Beat the egg
- Put soya mince into a bowl, add fennel seeds, milk, breadcrumbs, pine nuts, sun-dried tomatoes, rosemary, oregano, cooled onion mixture & beaten egg & mix thoroughly
- Spoon mixture into a small oven proof dish or ramekin (one that holds approx. 300 ml)
- Press down well & evenly & bake in oven for 1 hour
- Meanwhile boil the potatoes & cook peas
- Transfer mince loaf to serving plate, cut into 3 slices & serve with the boiled potatoes and peas
- Garnish with parsley & enjoy!

Speedy Cassoulet

Ingredients

1-cal cooking spray
1 small garlic clove, crushed
1 small onion, chopped
¼ fennel bulb, chopped
1 small carrot, peeled & chopped
200g tinned chopped tomatoes
1tsp dried thyme
112g canned cannellini beans, drained
100g canned pinto beans, drained
2 tsp tomato puree
freshly ground black pepper
75g Quom (chicken-style) pieces
few sprigs chopped fresh parsley
Tabasco sauce
60g couscous (dry weight)

Method

- Spray a non-stick saucepan with cooking spray & heat
- Fry garlic, onion, fennel & carrot for 2 minutes
- Add tomatoes, thyme, beans, tomato puree, pepper & bring to the boil

- Lower heat to medium & continue cooking, uncovered, for approx. 10 minutes
- Add Quorn pieces & heat for 1-2 minutes, stirring continuously
- Add a splash of Tabasco sauce (optional)
- Serve with a bowl of couscous (cooked to instructions on packaging) & garnish with parsley

Veggie Goulash

Ingredients

1-cal olive oil
¼ medium onion, thinly sliced
56g Quorn pieces
1 small green pepper, thinly sliced
½ teaspoon paprika
½ clove garlic, chopped
200g canned chopped tomatoes with juice
½ teaspoon dried oregano
½ teaspoon tomato puree
60ml red wine
pinch of stevia
ground black pepper

Method

- Coat frying pan with 8 sprays olive oil over medium heat
- Fry onion until tender, then add Quorn & green pepper
- Cook for further 5 minutes, stirring continuously until pepper is tender
- Stir in paprika and garlic
- Add tomatoes and juice and stir well
- Mix in oregano and tomato puree and stir in wine

- Bring to boil, reduce heat, cover and simmer for 20 minutes, stirring occasionally
- When liquid is thickened, stir in stevia & pepper
- Serve immediately.

Sweet Potato with Spicy Lentils & Coleslaw

Ingredients

1 medium sweet potato

2 tsp rapeseed oil

1 small onion, sliced finely

2 cm piece fresh ginger, peeled & grated

1 garlic clove, crushed

1 tsp ground cumin

1 tsp ground coriander

1 small green chilli, finely chopped (deseeded if you don't like it too hot)

200ml water

40g split red lentils

1 tsp zest lemon

1 tbsp lemon juice

¼ small pack coriander, chopped & couple of sprigs for garnish)

1 medium tomato, chopped

Coleslaw

1 tbsp extra virgin olive oil

1 tsp lemon juice

freshly ground black pepper

100g red cabbage, sliced finely

1 spring onion, sliced finely

1 small carrot, peeled & grated

1 tsp mixed seeds

2 tsp sultanas

Method

- Preheat oven to 220^{0}C
- Place potato on a baking tray & bake for approx. 40 minutes (until soft)
- Meanwhile, heat oil in non-stick, lidded frying pan
- Fry onion, stirring continuously for 3-5 minutes (until golden brown)
- Add ginger, garlic, cumin, coriander & chilli & cook for a few seconds, whilst stirring
- Add in lentils pour over 200ml water, stir thoroughly & bring to the boil
- Add lemon zest & lemon juice, stir well and reduce the heat to low
- Cover pan loosely & simmer for approx. 20 minutes (until the lentils are tender) stirring occasionally
- Mix in chopped coriander & tomatoes & cook for another 5 minutes, stirring constantly.
- If lentils thicken over much, add a dash of water
- Sprinkle with pepper, to taste
- To create the coleslaw - combine oil & lemon juice in a bowl, season with pepper
- Add cabbage, onion carrot, sultanas & seeds & mix thoroughly

- Put potato on serving plate, halve it & spoon lentils over
- Garnish with coriander and enjoy with your homemade coleslaw

Leek - Style Linguine

Ingredients

1 large leek, shredded
2 tsp butter
15ml white wine
2 tbsp crème fraîche
100g linguine
freshly ground pepper
1 tsp reduced fat cheddar cheese
squeeze of lemon juice

Method

- Put leeks with 1 tsp butter in a pan & stir gently over low heat
- Stir in remaining butter & white wine & cook gently for 5 minutes
- Add in crème fraîche & cook for approx. 15 minutes (until leeks are soft)
- Season with pepper, to taste
- Cook the pasta according to instructions on packet
- Mix in the leek mixture & transfer to plate
- Top with cheese & squeeze of lemon juice

Spicy Pasta Squash & Cottage Cheese

Ingredients

125g dried pasta

150g ready-to-use butternut squash

1-cal cooking spray

½ tsp cumin seeds

¼ tsp dried red chilli flakes

50g baby spinach leaves

50g low fat natural cottage cheese

freshly ground black pepper

lettuce leaves

Method

- Put pasta & squash into a pan of boiling water for approx. 12 minutes (until squash is soft & pasta is cooked)
- Drain except for 3 tablespoons of the cooking water, which is tipped into a cup
- Coat a non-stick frying pan with cooking spray & heat gently
- Stir in cumin seeds & chilli flakes & fry for 30 seconds
- Add the pasta, squash, spinach leaves & remaining cooking liquid

- Stir the mixture & cook on a low heat for 2 minutes (until the spinach wilts)
- Take the pan off the heat & stir in cottage cheese
- Add pepper to season & mix well
- Serve with a bowl of crisp lettuce

Perfect Pasta, Beans, Pepper & Onions

Ingredients

28g wholewheat spaghetti

1 tsp olive oil

1 clove garlic, crushed

112g frozen peppers & onions

small can cannellini beans, rinsed & drained

1 tbsp dry white wine

1 tsp lemon juice

pinch of dried crushed thyme

freshly ground black pepper

pinch of cayenne pepper

1 tsp olive oil spread

½ tsp lemon zest

Method

- Cook pasta according to directions on package
- Meanwhile, heat oil in frying pan on medium heat
- Stir in garlic & cook for about 20 seconds
- Stir in the frozen vegetables & cook for 2 minutes
- Add in beans, wine, lemon juice, thyme , black pepper, cayenne pepper & bring to the boil

- Turn heat down low & simmer gently, stirring occasionally, for approx. 4 minutes (until vegetables are tender)
- Remove from heat & stir in olive oil spread
- Drain the pasta & combine it with the vegetables in the frying pan
- Spoon pasta mixture into a bowl & top with lemon zest

Spicy Tofu with Barley Pilaf

Ingredients

200ml vegetable stock

60g pearl barley

½ tsp ground cinnamon

½ tsp ground cumin

pinch of white pepper

4 tsp rapeseed oil

75g firm tofu, sliced

2 cm fresh ginger root, finely chopped

1 clove garlic, crushed

¼ tsp Chinese 5-spice (salt & sugar free)

60g onion, finely sliced

80g yellow pepper, chopped finely

80g red pepper, chopped finely

70g courgette, diced

50g frozen peas, defrosted

40g pomegranate seeds

1 tsp reduced-salt soy sauce

12g fresh chopped coriander

Method

- Put stock, barley, cinnamon, cumin & pepper into a saucepan on a medium-high heat & bring to the boil
- Reduce heat, cover & simmer for 20 minutes
- Stir so that it does not stick & if necessary cook for a few minutes longer until tender, then remove from heat
- Meanwhile, put 2 tsp of the oil in a non-stick frying pan & tofu slices for approx. 5 minutes on each side (until golden brown)
- Remove tofu from the pan to let them cool slightly before slicing into smaller pieces
- Put ginger & garlic in the frying pan & cook for 1-2 minutes
- Return the cooked tofu to the pan, sprinkle with 5-spice, mix well & remove from the heat
- Put the remaining 2 tsp oil in another pan & heat gently
- Add onion, peppers & courgette & cook for 5 minutes, stirring continuously (until soft)
- Mix peas & prepared barley into cooked vegetables
- Spoon onto plate, top with tofu, pomegranate seeds & soy sauce
- Garnish with coriander
- Eat whilst deliciously hot or leave until later to eat cold – a tasty dish whichever way you choose to consume it!

Penne with Asparagus

Ingredients

125g dried penne pasta

1-cal cooking spray

1 small garlic clove, crushed

90g asparagus, trimmed & halved

freshly ground black pepper

50g frozen peas

100g cherry tomatoes

50ml hot vegetable stock

6 fresh basil leaves, chopped

Method

- Cook the pasta following packet instructions, drain & reserve 2 tbsp of the cooking water
- Meanwhile, coat a non-stick frying pan with cooking spray heat gently; add the garlic cook, whilst stirring for 30 seconds
- Mix in the asparagus, season with pepper & stir-fry for 3 minutes (until softened)
- Add peas & tomatoes & cook for 2 minutes
- Pour in the stock & heat until mixture simmers
- Continue cooking for approx. 5 minutes (until the tomatoes split & the stock is reduced by half)

- Spoon mixture into a serving bowl
- Stir the pasta in well, adding reserved cooking to loosen the pasta
- Gently stir in the chopped basil
- It's ready to eat!

Quinoa & Vegetable

Ingredients

150 ml water

63g quinoa

2 tsp olive oil

1 small onion, chopped

1 small potato, chopped

1 small stick celery, chopped

1 small courgette, chopped

½ red chilli, finely chopped

½ tsp ground coriander

½ tsp ground cumin

200g can chopped tomatoes

½ tsp dried oregano

freshly ground black pepper

15g walnuts, chopped

Method

- Pour 300ml of water into a saucepan & bring to the boil
- Add quinoa & simmer for approx. 10-15 minutes until all water is absorbed & then remove from heat
- Heat oil in a non-stick frying pan & cook onion for

3-4 minutes (until softened)
- Stir in potato, celery & courgette & continue to cook for a further 5 minutes
- Stir in chilli, coriander & cumin & cook for another minute
- Add tomatoes, oregano & black pepper to taste & simmer for 10–15 minutes, until the vegetables are cooked through
- Stir in the quinoa and walnuts
- Serve while hot

Veggie Pasta

Ingredients

30g wholemeal dried pasta shapes

1 tbsp olive oil

½ onion, finely chopped

1 small carrot, diced

½ small yellow pepper, chopped

125ml reduced-salt vegetable stock

¼ heaped tsp dried oregano

1 small cabbage leaf, chopped

12g edamame beans

½ tsp pesto

ground black pepper

Method

- Put pasta into a saucepan of boiling water, cook for 8 minutes before draining & putting to one side
- Meanwhile, heat oil gently in a frying a pan & stir in the onion, carrot & yellow pepper
- Cook for approx. 5 minutes (until mixture begins to brown)
- Pour in stock, stir in oregano & bring to the boil
- Lower the heat, add cabbage & beans & cook until

mixture begins to boil (approx 2 minutes), stirring regularly
- Add pasta, bring to boiling point before removing from the heat
- Transfer to a bowl & add pesto
- Sprinkle generously with black pepper & eat slowly

Tasty Risotto

Ingredients

1 tbsp olive oil

2 spring onions, chopped

450ml low salt vegetable stock

1 small clove garlic, crushed

Small pinch white pepper

75g brown risotto rice

100g asparagus tips

75g frozen peas, defrosted

1 tsp half-fat crème fraîche

1 tsp butter

5g low fat cheddar cheese, grated

Method

- Put oil into a heavy-based saucepan
- Stir in spring onions & cook for 1 minute over medium heat
- Heat stock in another saucepan & keep simmering gently
- Add garlic & white pepper to the onions & stir for 1 minute
- Stir in rice & cook for 2 more minutes
- Add approx. two ladles of stock (to just cover the

rice) & stir
- Regularly stir the rice, adding hot stock a little at a time over a 20 minutes period, so the rice is just covered & risotto is bubbling very gently
- At end of 20 minutes, add any remaining stock, peas & asparagus tips
- Cook for 2 -5 minutes (until rice is slightly firm)
- Remove from heat, stir in crème fraiche, butter & cheese. Cover and leave for 2 minutes before serving

Barbequed Sweet Potato, Feta & Fennel Parcel

Ingredients

1 sweet potato, peeled & cut into wedges
½ small fennel bulb, sliced
1 tbsp olive oil
1 tbsp orange juice
1 tsp of orange zest
2 tsp red wine vinegar
1 tbsp chopped parsley
1 tsp runny honey
ground black pepper
1 tbsp chopped walnuts
50g feta cheese, crumbled

Method

- Put potato wedges & fennel onto the centre of a 30cm square piece of cooking foil
- Coat with mixture of 1 tsp of the oil & 1 tsp of the orange juice
- Fold foil up around the veg & scrunch top to form a sealed parcel
- Put the parcel on the rack over the hottest part of barbecue
- Bake for 35-45 mins until potato is soft (Unwrap

and test with the point of a knife to make sure it's cooked)
- Meanwhile, make dressing by whisking together the remaining 2 tsp orange juice & oil with vinegar, parsley, honey, walnuts & zest
- Sprinkle with pepper
- When the potato is cooked remove it carefully from the heat, open the top of the parcel, stir in the dressing & the feta cheese & eat while warm

Spicy Rice with Raita

Ingredients

4 tsp rapeseed oil

45g brown basmati rice

1 tsp ground coriander

½ tsp ground turmeric

seeds from 3 cardamom pods

1 bay leaf

2 tsp finely chopped fresh ginger

½ red chilli, deseeded & chopped finely

12g creamed coconut, chopped

100g can chickpeas (undrained)

1 small pepper, chopped

100g cauliflower florets, broken into small pieces

1 small onion, sliced

¼ tsp cumin seeds

Raita

75ml pot natural fat free yogurt

1 tbsp cucumber, chopped finely

8g mint leaves, chopped

Method

- Preheat oven to 220°C
- Meanwhile put 2 tsp of rapeseed oil in non-stick, lidded frying pan & heat gently
- Add rice & sauté with coriander, turmeric, cardamom seeds, bay leaf, ginger and chilli
- Pour in 160ml water and add creamed coconut
- Bring to the boil, cover the pan & simmer for 15 mins
- Stir in chickpeas (with their liquid) & cook, covered, for a further 10 minutes
- In a bowl mix the remaining 2 tsp oil with red pepper, cauliflower, and onion in the oil & cumin seeds
- Transfer mixture to a baking sheet in oven & roast for 20 mins (until veg is tender)
- During the time the rice & veg are cooking make raita - mix together yogurt, cucumber & half of the chopped mint
- Once veg & rice are tender (with the stock absorbed), mix everything together & scoop onto serving plate
- Scatter rest of mint over and serve with a small side dish of raita

Chargrilled Vegetable Pasta

Ingredients

125g wholemeal pasta
½ small aubergine, diced
½ courgette, diced
½ small red pepper, deseeded & diced
½ small yellow pepper, deseeded & diced
½ small red onion, chopped
1 small garlic clove, crushed
freshly ground black pepper
1-cal cooking oil spray
50g passata with onion and garlic
2 tsp of fresh basil, shredded

Method

- Cook the pasta according to the packet instructions, drain and put to one side
- Preheat grill to medium-high
- Place aubergine, courgette, peppers, onion & garlic on a grill pan, sprinkle with pepper to taste & mix
- Spray 3 times with the oil over the mix
- Grill for approx 8 minutes (until softened), turning the vegetables frequently

- Meanwhile, heat passata for approx. 1 minute in a saucepan on medium heat
- Mix grilled vegetables into the passata & stir well to coat them thoroughly
- Stir vegetables mix into the pasta
- Scoop onto serving plate
- Garnish with basil

Spicy Sweet Chickpea Rice

Ingredients

75g dried long-grain brown rice

100g can chickpeas, drained

juice & grated zest of ½ lime

tiny pinch of stevia

¼ tsp cumin seeds

1 tsp curry powder

¼ tsp dried mint

½ tsp dried coriander

1-cal cooking spray

1 small red onion, sliced

1 small red pepper, deseeded & sliced

100g baby plum tomatoes, halved

Method

- Cook rice following instructions on packet, drain & cover to keep warm
- Meanwhile, put chickpeas into a bowl & stir in the lime juice & zest, stevia, cumin seeds, curry powder, mint & coriander
- Coat a non-stick frying pan with the cooking spray, heat gently, add onion, stir continuously for approx. 3 minutes or until just beginning to brown

- Turn down heat to medium, add peppers & cook for 3 minutes (until vegetables are tender) stirring from time to time
- Add tomatoes, chickpea mixture & cooked rice
- Cook for approx 2 minutes (until completely heated through)
- Transfer to a plate & enjoy!

Veggie Stew

Ingredients

1 tbsp olive oil

1 small onion, sliced

150ml vegetable stock

¼ tsp yeast extract

1 tbsp tomato puree

1 potato, peeled & chopped

1 carrot, peeled & chopped

1 stick celery, chopped

56g mushrooms, sliced

56g cauliflower florets

1 small parsnip, peeled & chopped

1 thumb-sized piece of swede, peeled & chopped

1 bay leaf

½ tsp mixed herbs

freshly ground pepper

crusty wholemeal roll or small bowl of mashed potato

Method

- Heat oil in pan & sauté onion until softened

- Boil stock & dissolve yeast extract in it & stir in tomato puree
- Add vegetables to saucepan with the stock & herbs
- Bring to the boil, cover & simmer for approx. 20–30 minutes (until tender)
- Season with pepper
- Enjoy with a crusty wholemeal roll or mashed potato

Sweet Potato Bake

Ingredients

1-cal olive oil spray
1 large sweet potato
1small avocado, peeled & de-stoned
juice of ½ lime
1 vine tomato, chopped finely
½ red chilli, deseeded & chopped finely
½ small red onion, finely chopped
small handful coriander, leaves, chopped
200g canned red kidney beans in water, drained
small wedge lime

Method

- Preheat oven to 220^{0}C
- Use 1 spray of oil on each side of the sweet potato
- Place potato on oven shelf & bake for approx. 45 minutes (until tender when pierced with knife)
- Meanwhile, mash avocado in a bowl with the lime juice
- Add the tomato, chilli, onion & coriander
- Cut potato in half
- Top with avocado mixture & beans
- Serve with lime wedge (to squeeze over)

Tasty Broccoli Pasta

Ingredients

½ broccoli head, trimmed & cut into florets

75g fusilli pasta

¼ tsp chilli flakes

2 small garlic cloves, crushed

1 tbsp crème fraîche

freshly ground pepper

2 tsp olive oil

28g feta cheese

Method

- Bring a medium saucepan of water (with a little salt added) to the boil
- Put in the broccoli & cook for 10 minutes before transferring, using a slotted spoon, into medium - sized bowl
- Cook the pasta in the same water following instructions on packet
- Meanwhile, mash broccoli before stirring in chilli flakes, garlic & crème fraîche & seasoning with pepper to taste
- Drain cooked pasta well & stir in the olive oil
- Crumble feta over the pasta & serve

Roasted Onion & Courgette with Spaghetti

Ingredients

I -cal olive oil cooking spray
½ medium onion, sliced thickly
1 medium courgette, sliced thickly
½ tsp ground black pepper
200g wholewheat spaghetti
1 tbsp low fat cheddar cheese, grated
plenty of green salad

Salad Dressing:

60ml olive oil
2 tbsp balsamic vinegar
1 tsp dried basil, ¼ tsp salt, ¼ tsp
ground pepper
1 small clove garlic (chopped)

Method

- Make dressing for salad by combining all the ingredients for it
- Drizzle over salad & toss lightly
- Preheat oven to 260^{0}C

- Cook spaghetti according to instructions on packet, drain & cover
- Use aluminium foil to line 2 large baking trays & spray with oil to coat
- Spread onion & courgette onto trays, sprinkle with pepper & cover lightly with oil spray
- Roast for 8 – 10 minutes (until vegetables are firm inside & tender outside)
- Mix vegetables into cooked spaghetti on serving plate
- Sprinkle cheese over
- Serve with prepared dressed salad - colourful & delicious!

Easy Cheesy Pasta

Ingredients

75g pasta

½ head, broccoli florets

1tbsp olive oil

½ tbsp pine nuts

½ clove garlic, sliced

50g low fat cheddar cheese, finely grated

Method

- Cook pasta according to instructions on packet & drain, reserving 1 tbsp cooking water
- In pan of boiling water, cook broccoli for 1-2 minutes
- Drain & chop finely
- Heat olive oil in non-stick frying pan & cook pine nuts & garlic for approx. 3 minutes
- Stir in broccoli to warm through
- Mix in drained pasta & the tbsp cooking water
- Add half the cheese & toss
- Serve, topped with the rest of the cheese

Rice Salad

Ingredients

1 tsp rapeseed oil

1 tsp sesame oil

1 tsp freshly grated ginger root

2 tsp low sodium soy sauce

2 tbsp rice vinegar

75g medium-grain rice, cooked according to instructions on packet & drained

½ small red onion, chopped finely

30g carrot, grated

125g cucumber, peeled & chopped finely

2 tsp sesame seeds

Method

- Mix the rapeseed & sesame oils with the ginger, soy sauce & vinegar in a small bowl
- Put cooked rice in a larger bowl
- Stir the mixture into the rice
- Add onion, carrot & cucumber
- Sprinkle sesame seeds over
- Serve with a happy face!

Pumpkin, Leek & Onion Quinoa

Ingredients

1 tbsp olive oil

1 medium leek, trimmed & sliced

150g pumpkin, diced

1 small onion, sliced finely

1 clove garlic, chopped

leaves of 2 sprigs of thyme

56g quinoa

1 tsp lemon juice

freshly ground pepper

1 tbsp parsley, chopped finely

2 tbsp pine nuts, toasted lightly

Method

- Cook pine nuts in a dry, non-stick frying pan, over a low heat for approx. 3 minutes, stirring frequently (until just golden brown) & then remove quickly from heat, to avoid burning
- Heat oil in another non-stick pan & add leek, pumpkin, onion, garlic & thyme
- Meanwhile rinse quinoa thoroughly in water
- Put quinoa into a different saucepan, cover completely with water & bring to the boil

- Turn heat to low & simmer for 10 minutes (until it is tender)
- Drain well & leave on one side in the saucepan, covered with a lid
- Once vegetables are cooked transfer them to a serving bowl & stir in the quinoa
- Mix in lemon juice, pepper, parsley & pine nuts before eating

Made in the USA
Monee, IL
31 August 2019